ULTIMATE PROPER BODY BUILDING

THE ESSENTIAL GUIDE TO STRENGTH, HEALTH AND CONFIDENCE

FRANK C. MOORE

CONTENTS

Chapter 1
Introduction

Overview of the 30-Day Program

Welcome to "A 30 Days Ultimate Proper Body Building," a transformative guide designed to propel you towards your fitness aspirations. In this opening chapter, we set the stage for a journey that extends beyond physical transformation; it's about embracing a lifestyle centered around proper bodybuilding.

Setting Realistic Goals

Before diving into the intricacies of the program, we emphasize the importance of setting realistic and achievable goals. Whether your aim is to build muscle, shed fat, or enhance overall fitness, clearly defined objectives serve as the compass that guides your efforts over the next 30 days.

Understanding the Philosophy

Holistic Approach to BodyBuilding

Unlike conventional approaches, our program adopts a holistic perspective on bodybuilding. It goes beyond the mere pursuit of muscle mass, encompassing aspects of nutrition, recovery, and mental resilience. The goal is not just a physical transformation but a sustainable and balanced lifestyle change.

The Science Behind 30 Days

We delve into the science behind the 30-day timeframe. While it may seem brief, this duration is strategically crafted to instill discipline, kickstart habits, and lay the foundation for long-term success. We explore the psychological and physiological aspects that make the next 30 days a pivotal period in your fitness journey.

Laying the Groundwork

Importance of Mindset

Before you embark on the physical journey, cultivating the right mindset is paramount. We discuss the power of positivity, resilience in the face of challenges, and how a strong mental foundation can amplify your physical gains.

Assessing Your Starting Point

Understanding where you are currently is crucial for progress. We guide you through self-assessment, helping you identify strengths, weaknesses, and areas for improvement. This introspection sets the stage for a tailored and effective 30-day plan.

Closing Thoughts

As you turn the pages of this guide, remember that this is not just a program; it's a commitment to your well-being. The next 30 days are an opportunity to redefine your relationship with fitness, nutrition, and self-discipline. So, fasten your seatbelt, embrace the challenge, and get ready for a holistic transformation that extends far beyond the physical realm.

Chapter 2

Understanding Body Types

Introduction to body typing

Embarking on a successful bodybuilding journey necessitates a profound understanding of your body type. In this chapter, we unravel the intricacies of the three primary body types—ectomorph, mesomorph, and endomorph—exploring how these genetic predispositions profoundly shape muscle development, metabolism, and overall physique.

Ectomorphs: The Hard Gainers

Ectomorphs, characterized by a slender and lean physique, often encounter challenges in gaining muscle mass. We delve into the nuances of their metabolism, providing comprehensive strategies that encompass high-calorie nutrition plans, specialized workout routines, and targeted supplementation to overcome the inherent difficulty in bulking up.

Mesomorphs: The Athletic Build

Mesomorphs, blessed with a naturally athletic build, possess a genetic advantage in muscle development. This section explores how mesomorphs can optimize their inherent strengths through tailored training techniques and nutrition plans. We aim to guide mesomorphs in achieving a balanced and sculpted physique.

Endomorphs: The Naturally Solid

Endomorphs, predisposed to store more fat, face unique challenges in achieving lean muscle gain. We provide an in-depth examination of dietary adjustments, high-intensity training, and metabolic considerations to enhance fat loss while simultaneously building muscle mass, fostering a healthier and more defined physique.

The Hybrid Body Types

Recognizing the complexity of individual physiques, we introduce the concept of hybrid body types, acknowledging that many individuals exhibit characteristics of more than one body type. This nuanced approach allows for a more personalized strategy, embracing the diversity inherent in human genetics.

Chapter 3

Basics of Nutrition

Introduction

In the realm of bodybuilding, the significance of nutrition cannot be overstated. Chapter 3 unfolds the essential principles that underscore a well-rounded approach to nutrition, illuminating the path toward optimal muscle growth, sustained energy, and overall well-being.

Importance of a Balanced Diet

The Fuel for Your Engine

Think of your body as a high-performance engine—nutrition is the fuel that propels it forward. We delve into the critical components of a balanced diet, emphasizing the role of macronutrients (proteins, carbohydrates, and fats) and micronutrients (vitamins and minerals). Understanding the synergy between these elements lays the foundation for a diet that supports your bodybuilding goals.

Timing and Portion Control

Beyond the composition of your meals, we explore the significance of meal timing and portion control. Tailoring your nutrient intake to match the demands of your workout routine optimizes energy levels, enhances recovery, and fuels the muscle-building process. Practical insights on portion sizes help strike the delicate balance between consuming enough calories for growth without unnecessary excess.

Nutrient-Rich Foods for Muscle Building

The Protein Puzzle

Protein is the cornerstone of muscle building, and we dissect its importance in detail. From complete and incomplete protein sources to the concept of protein synthesis, this section guides you in making informed choices that elevate your protein intake. Whether it's lean meats, plant-based proteins, or supplements, we navigate the diverse landscape of protein options.

Carbohydrates as Energy Currency

Your body uses carbohydrates as its main energy source, particularly during vigorous exercise. We explore complex and simple carbohydrates, emphasizing their role in replenishing glycogen stores and sustaining energy levels. Practical strategies for incorporating carbohydrates into your diet ensure a well-rounded and sustainable energy source.

Fats: The Unsung Hero

Dispelling myths about fats, we highlight their crucial role in hormone production and overall health. By distinguishing between healthy fats and their counterparts, you gain the knowledge to integrate fats strategically into your diet. This section offers a nuanced approach that goes beyond mere calorie counting.

Hydration and Its Impact

The Overlooked Elixir

Amidst discussions of macronutrients, the significance of hydration often takes a back seat. We delve into the multifaceted benefits of staying adequately hydrated, from supporting metabolic processes to promoting recovery. Practical tips on maintaining optimal fluid balance complement your nutritional strategy.

Creating Your Nutrition Plan

Tailoring Nutrition to Your Body Type

Building on insights from Chapter 2, we align nutritional recommendations with specific body types. Whether you're an ectomorph requiring surplus calories or an endomorph aiming for a controlled intake, this section offers practical guidelines to customize your nutrition plan.

Meal Prepping and Planning

Success in bodybuilding often hinges on preparation. We guide you through the art of meal prepping and planning, empowering you to navigate busy schedules while ensuring consistent adherence to your nutritional goals. From grocery lists to batch cooking, these practical tips foster a seamless integration of your nutrition plan into your lifestyle.

Supplement Guidance

Enhancing, Not Replacing

While supplements can complement your nutrition plan, they should not serve as substitutes for whole foods. We demystify the world of supplements, providing insights into when and how to incorporate them effectively. From protein powders to vitamins, you gain a nuanced understanding of supplementation as a supportive element in your bodybuilding journey.

Adapting Your Nutrition Plan

The Dynamic Nature of Nutrition

Just as your body evolves, so should your nutrition plan. We explore strategies for adapting your dietary approach based on progress, goals, and lifestyle changes. This forward-thinking perspective ensures that your nutrition plan remains a dynamic and sustainable component of your bodybuilding journey.

Conclusion

Chapter 3 serves as a nutritional compass, guiding you through the intricate terrain of fueling your body for optimal performance and growth. Armed with knowledge about balanced diets, nutrient-rich foods, and strategic supplementation, you are poised to embark on the next 30 days with a nutrition plan that not only supports your bodybuilding goals but becomes an integral part of a holistic, healthy lifestyle.

Chapter 4

Creating Your Workout Plan

Introduction

Welcome to the heart of your transformative journey—Chapter 4: Creating Your Workout Plan. This section is the architectural blueprint that will guide you through 30 days of intentional, effective, and goal-oriented workouts. As we delve into the intricacies of structuring your training regimen, keep in mind that your workout plan is more than a series of exercises; it's a carefully crafted roadmap to sculpting your physique.

Weekly Breakdown of Exercises

Strategic Organization

We begin by dissecting the week into strategically organized segments, each dedicated to specific muscle groups. Mondays may be devoted to chest and triceps, Tuesdays to back and biceps, and so forth. This approach ensures a comprehensive and balanced engagement of your musculature, allowing for optimal growth and recovery.

Progressive Overload Principles

Central to our 30-day program is the principle of progressive overload. This means systematically increasing the demands on your muscles over time. We discuss various techniques—from adjusting weights to manipulating repetitions—ensuring that your muscles are consistently challenged. This dynamic approach keeps your body adapting and growing throughout the program.

Balancing Cardio and Strength Training

An often-overlooked aspect of bodybuilding is the integration of cardiovascular exercise. We explore the symbiotic relationship between cardio and strength training, outlining how they complement each other. High-Intensity Interval Training (HIIT) and steady-state cardio find their place in your weekly routine, fostering not only muscle development but also cardiovascular health.

Perfecting Form and Technique

The Foundation of Progress

The effectiveness of any workout hinges on proper form and technique. We delve into the intricacies of key exercises, emphasizing the importance of correct execution. From squats to bench presses, mastering these fundamental movements not only maximizes muscle engagement but also mitigates the risk of injuries.

Common Mistakes to Avoid

Knowledge is power, and understanding common pitfalls is crucial. We highlight frequent mistakes individuals make during workouts and provide guidance on how to sidestep them. This section acts as a preemptive strike against potential setbacks, ensuring your 30-day journey is marked by progress rather than impediments.

Rest and Recovery

Importance of Rest Days

The saying "muscles are built during rest" is accurate. We emphasize the significance of incorporating rest days into your program. Rest is not a sign of weakness but a strategic element in the muscle-building process. We guide you in understanding when and how to integrate rest days for optimal recovery.

Techniques for Effective Recovery

Recovery extends beyond mere rest days. We explore techniques such as stretching, foam rolling, and adequate sleep that contribute to effective recovery. Understanding the holistic nature of recuperation ensures that your body is primed for each successive workout, minimizing the risk of burnout or overtraining.

Monitoring Progress

Tracking Fitness Metrics

Measurement is a powerful motivator. We discuss the importance of tracking key fitness metrics—strength gains, changes in body composition, and overall performance. These tangible markers not only validate your efforts but also provide valuable insights for making informed adjustments to your plan.

Adjusting the Plan Based on Results

Flexibility is a cornerstone of success. As you progress through the 30 days, we guide you on how to interpret your results and make necessary adjustments. Whether it's increasing weights, tweaking exercises, or modifying the overall structure, adapting your plan based on real-time feedback ensures continued growth and prevents plateaus.

Motivation and Discipline

Staying Committed to the Program

Motivation waxes and wanes, but discipline is a constant. We discuss strategies for staying committed to the program, from setting short-term goals to finding a workout buddy. Cultivating discipline transforms your workout plan from a 30-day sprint into a sustainable fitness journey.

Overcoming Challenges and Setbacks

Obstacles are unavoidable, but how you overcome them determines your level of success. We provide practical tools for overcoming setbacks, whether they be time constraints, fatigue, or unforeseen obstacles. Resilience is the bedrock of long-term fitness success.

Conclusion

Chapter 4 is more than a manual for lifting weights; it's your companion in the pursuit of physical excellence. Your workout plan is not a static entity; it's a living, breathing guide that evolves with you. As you embark on the next 30 days, remember that every rep, every set, and every rest day is a brick in the foundation of your success. Stay consistent, stay focused, and let the next 30 days mark the beginning of a stronger, fitter, and more resilient you.

Chapter 5

Perfecting Form and Technique

Introduction

Welcome to the pivotal chapter dedicated to the fine art of perfecting form and technique in your workouts. In the pursuit of an effective and injury-free bodybuilding journey, mastering the intricacies of each exercise is paramount. This chapter focuses on dissecting fundamental exercises, ensuring proper form and technique to optimize muscle engagement and safeguard against potential injuries.

The Foundation of Progress

Mastering Proper Form

The foundation of any successful workout is proper form. We delve into key exercises, providing clear explanations and visual guides to ensure correct execution. Mastering the mechanics of each movement guarantees efficient muscle targeting, fostering progress while minimizing the risk of injury.

Core Engagement and Stability

A strong core is the linchpin of proper form. We explore the role of core engagement in exercises, offering practical tips and exercises to enhance core strength. A stable core not only safeguards against injury but also boosts overall strength and performance.

Common Mistakes to Avoid

Addressing Spinal Alignment

Improper spinal alignment is a common pitfall. We tackle issues like overarching and underarching during exercises, providing visual cues and corrections to maintain a neutral spine. Ensuring correct spinal alignment safeguards your back and contributes to the effectiveness of the workout.

Perfecting Joint Alignment and Range of Motion

Accurate joint alignment and sufficient range of motion are imperative. We address common errors such as inadequate depth in squats or improper elbow positioning in various exercises. Understanding optimal joint mechanics enhances the effectiveness of each movement and reduces strain on joints.

Movement Patterns and Muscle Engagement

Maximizing Compound Movements

Understanding movement patterns is crucial for compound exercises. We break down the mechanics of squats, deadlifts, and bench presses, highlighting muscle engagement. This knowledge ensures that each repetition contributes to comprehensive muscle development.

Precision in Isolation Exercises

Isolation exercises demand precision. We provide detailed breakdowns of exercises like bicep curls and leg extensions, focusing on muscle isolation and correct form. Perfecting isolation exercises enhances targeted muscle growth.

Breathing Techniques

Rhythmic Breathing for Optimal Performance

Proper breathing is a often-overlooked aspect of effective workouts. We discuss the importance of rhythmic breathing during resistance training, syncing breath with movement to optimize oxygen supply. This section provides practical techniques for improved endurance and recovery.

Mobility and Flexibility

Dynamic Warm-Up for Improved Mobility

Mobility and flexibility are integral. We introduce dynamic warm-up routines that go beyond static stretching, preparing muscles and joints for resistance training. Improved mobility enhances range of motion and reduces the risk of injuries.

Corrective Exercises for Muscle Balance

Addressing muscular imbalances is paramount. We incorporate corrective exercises targeting areas prone to weaknesses or asymmetries. By rectifying imbalances, you ensure symmetrical muscle development and a resilient physique.

Incorporating Tempo and Eccentric Training

The Strategic Use of Tempo

Tempo training adds a new dimension to workouts. We explore how manipulating the speed of exercises influences muscle activation and growth. Incorporating tempo variations introduces a dynamic element to your training routine.

Unlocking Muscle Growth Through Eccentric Training

Eccentric training, emphasizing the lengthening phase of an exercise, is a powerful tool. We guide you through eccentric-focused exercises, outlining benefits and integration. Mastery of the eccentric component stimulates muscle growth.

Advanced Techniques for Form Mastery

Cultivating the Mind-Muscle Connection

The mind-muscle connection is transformative. We delve into the psychological aspect of training, teaching you to consciously engage specific muscles during exercises. Heightened awareness enhances muscle recruitment for a more effective workout.

Leveraging Video Analysis and Feedback

In the digital age, video analysis is a valuable tool. We discuss how recording and reviewing workouts provide insights into form and technique. Seeking feedback contributes to continual improvement, creating a feedback loop for ongoing progress.

Form Maintenance Across Various Training Modalities

Mastery in Bodyweight Exercises

Form maintenance extends to bodyweight exercises. We guide you through proper form in exercises like push-ups and pull-ups, ensuring mastery of fundamental movements.

Precision in Machine and Cable Exercises

Machines and cable systems introduce specific challenges. We guide you through adjusting machine settings, maintaining stability, and optimizing form. This section broadens your exercise repertoire for a diversified training experience.

Troubleshooting Form Challenges

Addressing Specific Concerns

Form challenges are part of the learning process. We provide a troubleshooting guide, addressing concerns such as grip strength, imbalances, and discomfort. Systematic solutions refine form, enhancing the overall effectiveness of your workouts.

Conclusion

Chapter 5 is your manual for refining every movement in your workout routine. Perfecting form and technique is an ongoing journey of improvement. As you embark on the next 30 days, treat each repetition as an opportunity to refine your skills, deepen your mind-muscle connection, and sculpt a physique that reflects not just strength, but mastery. Every precise movement contributes to the canvas of your

body's masterpiece—make each one deliberate
and purposeful.

CHAPTER 6

Rest and Recovery in Bodybuilding: A Comprehensive Guide

In the demanding realm of bodybuilding, where intensity and dedication are paramount, the often-underestimated pillars of rest and recovery play a pivotal role in achieving optimal results. This comprehensive guide delves into the intricacies of these essential components, exploring their significance, the physiological processes involved, and effective strategies for maximizing their benefits.

The Physiology of Rest and Recovery

Muscle Repair and Growth

After intense workouts, muscles experience microscopic damage. It is during the subsequent periods of rest that the body initiates repair processes. This repair not only addresses the damage but also leads to muscle growth, making adequate rest fundamental for building strength and size.

Hormonal Balance

Proper rest is crucial for maintaining hormonal equilibrium. Hormones like cortisol, associated with stress, and growth hormone, vital for muscle development, require a delicate balance.

Consistent and quality sleep, a key component of recovery, contributes significantly to hormonal regulation.

Neurological Recovery

Intense training places stress on the central nervous system. Sufficient rest allows for neurological recovery, ensuring optimal coordination, focus, and reaction times during workouts.

Prevention of Overtraining

Overtraining, a state of prolonged and excessive physical stress without adequate recovery, can lead to diminished performance, fatigue, and an increased risk of injuries. Scheduled rest days act as a preventative measure against the pitfalls of overtraining.

Importance of Rest Days

Microtrauma Repair

Rest days are not synonymous with inactivity; rather, they are strategic periods for the body to repair microtrauma within muscle fibers. This repair process contributes significantly to muscle hypertrophy and overall strength gains.

Psychological Rejuvenation

Beyond the physiological benefits, rest days provide an opportunity for psychological rejuvenation. A well-rested mind is better equipped to tackle subsequent workouts with focus and determination.

Preventing Burnout

Bodybuilding is a long-term endeavor, and burnout is a real concern for those pushing their limits. Strategic rest days interspersed throughout the training plan act as safeguards against mental and physical burnout.

Techniques for Effective Recovery

Quality Sleep

Quality sleep is the cornerstone of effective recovery. During the deep sleep stages, the body releases growth hormone, facilitating muscle repair and overall restoration. Aim for 7-9 hours of uninterrupted sleep each night.

Nutrition and Hydration

Post-exercise nutrition plays a critical role in recovery. Adequate protein intake, along with replenishing glycogen stores through carbohydrates, supports muscle repair. Staying well-hydrated is equally crucial for optimal metabolic function.

Active Recovery

Incorporating active recovery days into the training plan involves engaging in low-intensity activities such as walking, swimming, or yoga. These activities enhance blood flow, alleviate muscle soreness, and contribute to overall flexibility.

Mobility and Flexibility Work

Including mobility and flexibility exercises aids in preventing stiffness and improving joint range of motion. Dynamic stretching and targeted mobility drills can be particularly effective in promoting pliability.

Massage and Self-Care

Massage and self-myofascial release techniques contribute to recovery by releasing muscle tension, improving circulation, and hastening the removal of metabolic waste products.

Periodization for Optimal Recovery

Structuring Training Phases

Incorporating periodization into the training plan involves structuring training phases with varying intensities and volumes. This systematic approach prevents staleness, optimizes recovery, and promotes long-term progress.

Cyclical Approach to Intensity

Alternating between periods of high intensity and lower-intensity training provides the body with necessary breaks while ensuring continued progress. This cyclical approach helps prevent overtraining and fosters sustained improvements.

Monitoring and Adapting

Regular Assessments

Frequent assessments of training progress and overall well-being are essential. Monitoring key metrics such as strength gains, endurance improvements, and changes in body composition provides valuable insights into the effectiveness of the current regimen.

Listening to the Body

Attuning to the body's signals is crucial. Fatigue, persistent soreness, and changes in motivation can indicate the need for additional rest or modifications to the training plan. Listening to these cues fosters a balanced and sustainable approach to bodybuilding.

Conclusion

In conclusion, the significance of rest and recovery in bodybuilding cannot be overstated. It is not a mere cessation of activity; rather, it is a strategic and integral part of the overall training process. By embracing rest and employing effective recovery strategies, bodybuilders can optimize their gains, prevent burnout, and ensure a sustainable and fulfilling journey toward their ultimate fitness goals.

CHAPTER 7

Monitoring Progress in Bodybuilding: A Comprehensive Exploration

Embarking on a bodybuilding journey involves more than lifting weights and following a nutrition plan. The ability to monitor progress systematically is a crucial aspect that empowers individuals to make informed decisions, adjust their approach, and stay motivated on the path to their fitness goals. This comprehensive exploration delves into the intricacies of monitoring progress, offering insights, examples, and effective strategies for this integral facet of bodybuilding.

Establishing Baseline Measurements

Example 1: Body Composition Analysis**

Initiate your progress tracking by conducting a body composition analysis. This involves assessing metrics such as body weight, body fat percentage, and muscle mass. Documenting these baseline measurements provides a clear starting point for your bodybuilding journey.

Example 2: Strength Assessments

For those focusing on strength gains, conduct baseline strength assessments. Measure the maximum weight you can lift for specific exercises or determine the number of repetitions you can perform at a certain weight. These benchmarks serve as reference points for evaluating progress.

Example 3: Endurance and Cardiovascular Assessments

If cardiovascular fitness is a priority, conduct assessments related to endurance and cardiovascular health. This might involve measuring running times, tracking distances covered, or assessing improvements in recovery heart rate post-exercise.

Utilizing Workout Logs and Journals

Example 1: Strength Training Log

Maintain a detailed strength training log that records each workout session. Include information such as exercises performed, sets, repetitions, and the amount of weight lifted. A strength training log allows you to track progressive overload and identify areas for improvement.

Example 2: Nutrition Journal

A nutrition journal can be invaluable for monitoring dietary habits. Record daily food intake, including macronutrient breakdowns. This journal provides insights into nutritional patterns, aiding adjustments to support specific bodybuilding goals.

Example 3: Mood and Energy Journal

Consider maintaining a mood and energy journal to assess how external factors impact your workouts. Note stress levels, sleep quality, and other variables. This qualitative data contributes to a holistic understanding of your overall well-being.

Assessing Performance Metrics

Example 1: Progress Photos

Progress photos offer a visual representation of physical changes over time. Take consistent photos from various angles to observe changes in muscle definition, size, and overall physique. This tangible evidence can be a powerful motivator.

Example 2: Fitness Assessments

Periodically conduct fitness assessments tailored to your specific goals. This might involve reassessing cardiovascular fitness, flexibility, or functional movement patterns. Fitness assessments provide a holistic view of your overall fitness level.

Example 3: Psychological Assessments

Incorporate psychological assessments into your monitoring routine. Use tools like self-assessment questionnaires to gauge motivation levels, mental well-being, and overall satisfaction with your bodybuilding journey. Mental resilience is a key component of sustained progress.

Recognizing Plateaus and Adjusting Strategies

Example 1: Strength Plateau

If you notice a plateau in strength gains despite consistent efforts, it might be time to reassess your training program. Introduce variations such as changes in exercises, rep ranges, or workout intensity to break through stagnation.

Example 2: Nutritional Plateau

Plateaus in body composition or weight loss can occur due to nutritional factors. Analyze your nutrition journal to identify areas for improvement. Adjust macronutrient ratios, caloric intake, or meal timing based on your specific goals.

Example 3: Lifestyle Adjustments

External factors, such as increased stress or changes in daily routines, can impact progress. If faced with challenges, consider adapting your bodybuilding plan to accommodate these changes. This might involve modifying workout schedules, incorporating additional rest days, or adjusting training volume.

Setting and Celebrating Goals

Example 1: Short-Term and Long-Term Goals

Establish a combination of short-term and long-term goals. Short-term goals could include achieving specific strength milestones or adhering to a nutrition plan for a designated period. Long-term goals might encompass overarching fitness achievements such as body composition transformations.

Example 2: Goal Celebration

Celebrate achievements along the way. Acknowledge hitting a new personal best, reaching a weight loss target, or successfully completing a challenging workout. Celebrating milestones reinforces a positive mindset and enhances motivation for continued progress.

Adapting to Periodization Principles

Example 1: Intensity Cycling

Incorporate intensity cycling into your training plan. This might involve alternating phases of high-intensity training with periods of lower-intensity or active recovery. Adapting your training approach based on periodization principles prevents staleness and optimizes recovery.

Example 2: Deload Weeks

Integrate deload weeks into your training cycle. These are designated weeks with reduced training volume or intensity to allow for enhanced recovery. Deload weeks prevent overtraining, mitigate fatigue, and contribute to long-term progress.

Regularly Assessing and Adjusting

Example 1: Monthly Assessments

Conduct comprehensive assessments on a monthly basis. Review all available data, including workout logs, measurements, and psychological assessments. Use this information to identify patterns, assess the effectiveness of your strategies, and make informed adjustments.

Example 2: Dynamic Goal Setting

Maintain a dynamic approach to goal setting. As you progress, your goals may evolve. Regularly revisit and refine your goals to align with your changing priorities and aspirations within the bodybuilding journey.

Conclusion: A Continuous Journey of Improvement**

Monitoring progress in bodybuilding is not a static process; it's a dynamic and continuous journey of improvement. Utilize a combination of quantitative and qualitative assessments, adapt to the principles of periodization, and celebrate achievements along the way

Tracking Fitness Metrics: A Guide to Informed Progress

Monitoring fitness metrics is a cornerstone of any successful bodybuilding or fitness journey. The ability to systematically track and analyze various metrics provides valuable insights into your progress, helping you make informed decisions, set realistic goals, and stay motivated.

This guide explores key fitness metrics, why they matter, and how to effectively track them.

1. Body Composition Metrics:

a. Body Weight:

- **Importance:** Provides a general indication of overall mass.

- **Tracking Tip:** Weigh yourself consistently, preferably at the same time of day and under similar conditions (e.g., before breakfast).

b. Body Fat Percentage:

- **Importance**: Reflects the proportion of fat mass to total body weight.

- **Tracking Tip:** Use calipers, bioelectrical impedance, or dual-energy X-ray absorptiometry (DEXA) for accurate measurements.

c. Muscle Mass:

- **Importance:** Indicates the amount of muscle tissue in the body.

- **Tracking Tip**: Regularly assess muscle mass through body composition assessments or specific measurements.

2. Strength and Performance Metrics:

a. One-Rep Max (1RM):

- **Importance:** Measures the maximum weight lifted for a specific exercise.

- **Tracking Tip:** Test 1RM periodically, adjusting your training based on improvements.

b. Repetitions Maximum (RM):

- **Importance**: Determines the maximum number of repetitions at a given weight.

- **Tracking Tip:** Track your ability to perform higher reps over time for a specific weight.

c. Training Volume:

- **Importance:** Reflects the total workload in a workout (sets × reps × weight).

- **Tracking Tip**: Log your training volume to ensure progressive overload and track changes over weeks.

3. Endurance and Cardiovascular Metrics:

a. Running Times and Distances:

- **Importance:** Measures improvements in cardiovascular fitness and endurance.

- **Tracking Tip**: Record running times, distances, or other cardiovascular activities regularly.

b. Heart Rate and Recovery:

- **Importance:** Reflects cardiovascular health and recovery ability.

- **Tracking Tip**: Monitor your heart rate during and after workouts, noting changes in recovery times.

c. Flexibility and Range of Motion:

- **Importance**: Assesses joint flexibility and mobility.

- **Tracking Tip:** Regularly perform flexibility exercises and note improvements in range of motion.

4. Nutritional Metrics:

a. Caloric Intake:

- **Importance:** Determines the number of calories consumed daily.

- **Tracking Tip**: Use nutrition apps or journals to log food intake and assess against your goals.

b. Macronutrient Ratios:

- **Importance:** Balancing proteins, fats, and carbohydrates is crucial for performance and body composition.

- **Tracking Tip:** Monitor macronutrient ratios to align with your fitness objectives.

c. Hydration Levels:

- **Importance:** Adequate hydration supports metabolic processes and overall well-being.

- **Tracking Tip**: Ensure regular water intake and adjust based on activity levels and climate.

5. Psychological Metrics:

a. Motivation Levels:

- **Importance**: Reflects your enthusiasm and drive for training.

- **Tracking Tip:** Regularly assess your motivation and adjust your routine to maintain engagement.

b. Mental Well-being:

- **Importance**: Mental health impacts overall fitness and performance.

- **Tracking Tip:** Monitor stress levels, sleep quality, and mood for holistic well-being.

c. Perceived Exertion:

- **Importance:** Subjective assessment of effort during workouts.

- **Tracking Tip:** Use rating scales to gauge perceived exertion and adjust intensity accordingly.

6. Regular Assessments and Adjustments:

a. Periodic Assessments:

- **Importance:** Regular evaluations provide a snapshot of progress.

- **Tracking Tip:** Conduct comprehensive assessments monthly, adjusting strategies based on results.

b. Goal Reassessments:

- **Importance**: Goals may evolve; reassess periodically for alignment.

- **Tracking Tip**: Dynamically set and adapt goals based on changing priorities and achievements.

c. Adaptive Training:

- **Importance**: Adjust training plans based on assessments and changing circumstances.

- **Tracking Tip**: Be flexible in modifying workouts, rest days, or intensity to optimize progress.

Conclusion: Empowering Your Fitness Journey

Tracking fitness metrics goes beyond mere data collection; it empowers you to understand your body, make informed decisions, and cultivate a sustainable and effective fitness routine. Whether it's body composition, performance, nutrition, or psychological aspects, a holistic approach to tracking metrics contributes to a well-rounded and successful fitness journey. Regular assessments and adjustments based on these metrics ensure that you stay on the path to achieving your ultimate fitness goals.

Adjusting the Plan Based on Results: A Strategic Approach to Continuous Improvement

In the dynamic landscape of fitness and bodybuilding, the ability to adapt and refine your plan based on tangible results is a fundamental element for sustained progress. This guide explores the importance of adjusting your fitness plan, provides examples of common scenarios, and offers strategies to optimize your training and achieve your goals.

1. Progress Assessment:

Scenario 1: Strength Plateau

- **Observation:** You notice a stagnation in your ability to lift heavier weights or increase the number of repetitions.

- **Adjustment Strategy:** Introduce variations in your workout routine, such as changing exercises, adjusting rep ranges, or incorporating new training techniques. Progressive overload remains key, but the specific stimuli can vary to break through plateaus.

Scenario 2: Insufficient Recovery

- **Observation:** Lingering muscle soreness, decreased performance, and a general feeling of fatigue persist.

- **Adjustment Strategy**: Prioritize recovery. Increase the frequency of rest days, ensure adequate sleep, and consider incorporating active recovery techniques. Adjust workout intensity or volume to allow for proper recuperation.

2. Nutritional Adjustments:

Scenario 1: Weight Loss Plateau

- **Observation**: Despite consistent efforts, weight loss has stalled.

- **Adjustment Strategy:** Review your caloric intake and expenditure. Adjust your calorie deficit by either reducing intake slightly or increasing activity levels. Pay attention to macronutrient ratios to support your goals effectively.

Scenario 2: Energy Deficiency

- **Observation:**Persistent low energy levels and compromised performance during workouts.

- **Adjustment Strategy:** Assess your caloric intake and ensure you are meeting your energy requirements. Consider adjusting macronutrient distribution to optimize energy availability. Quality nutrition is crucial for sustained performance.

3. Adaptations for Overtraining:

Scenario 1: Decreased Performance

- **Observation:** A decline in strength, endurance, and overall workout performance.

- **Adjustment Strategy:** Implement a deload week to reduce training volume and intensity. Focus on recovery strategies, including adequate sleep, nutrition, and perhaps incorporating activities like yoga or light cardio for active recovery.

Scenario 2: Persistent Fatigue

- **Observation:** Lingering fatigue and a lack of enthusiasm for workouts.

- **Adjustment Strategy**: Reevaluate your training frequency, intensity, and duration. Adjust workout splits or consider strategic rest days. Prioritize quality over quantity to prevent burnout.

4. Goal-Specific Adjustments:

Scenario 1: Muscle Hypertrophy Focus
- **Observation**: Desire for increased muscle size and definition.
- **Adjustment Strategy:** Modify your training program to include higher-volume, hypertrophy-focused workouts. Adjust rep ranges, incorporate isolation exercises, and ensure a slight caloric surplus for optimal muscle growth.

Scenario 2: Endurance Improvement Goal
- **Observation**: Aiming for enhanced cardiovascular fitness and stamina.
- **Adjustment Strategy:** Incorporate more cardiovascular exercises into your routine. Adjust training ratios to include both high-intensity interval training (HIIT) and

steady-state cardio for a well-rounded endurance program.

5. Periodization Principles:

Scenario 1: Plateau Prevention
- **Observation:** Aiming to avoid plateaus and staleness in your routine.
- **Adjustment Strategy:** Implement periodization principles. Alternate between phases of high intensity and lower intensity. Periodically reassess your training plan to introduce new challenges and prevent adaptation plateaus.

Scenario 2: Goal-Specific Phases
- **Observation:** Pursuing diverse fitness goals within a yearly timeframe.
- **Adjustment Strategy:** Plan your training in phases. Allocate specific periods for strength building, hypertrophy, endurance, or skill development. This ensures a well-rounded and

periodized approach, preventing monotony and optimizing progress.

Conclusion: A Dynamic Fitness Journey

Adapting your fitness plan based on results is not a sign of failure but a strategic approach to continuous improvement. Regularly assess your progress, stay attuned to your body's signals, and be proactive in making adjustments. Whether breaking through plateaus, refining nutrition, preventing overtraining, or aligning with specific goals, the ability to adapt your plan ensures a dynamic and fulfilling fitness journey. Embrace the evolution, celebrate achievements, and persistently refine your approach for sustained success.

CHAPTER 8

Motivation and Discipline: Nurturing Commitment Through Challenges

Embarking on a fitness journey requires a delicate balance of motivation and discipline. While motivation sparks the initial drive, it's discipline that sustains commitment through challenges and setbacks. This guide explores strategies to cultivate motivation, build discipline, and overcome obstacles on the path to your fitness goals.

1. Cultivating Motivation:

a. Define Your "Why":

- **Strategy:** Clearly articulate your reasons for pursuing fitness. Whether it's improved health, enhanced performance, or a transformative physique, a well-defined "why" becomes a powerful source of intrinsic motivation.

b. Set SMART Goals:

- **Strategy:** Establish Specific, Measurable, Achievable, Relevant, and Time-bound (SMART) goals. Break down larger objectives into smaller, actionable steps to maintain focus and foster a sense of accomplishment.

c. Visualize Success:

- **Strategy**: Create a vivid mental image of your desired outcomes. Visualization can reinforce motivation by making your goals more tangible and exciting.

2. Building Discipline:

a. Establish Consistent Habits:

- **Strategy**: Create a routine that aligns with your fitness goals. Consistency builds discipline over time, making it easier to adhere to your program.

b. Prioritize and Schedule:

- **Strategy**: Prioritize your workouts and schedule them as non-negotiable appointments. Treat your fitness commitment with the same importance as other obligations in your life.

c. Accountability Systems:

- **Strategy**: Engage in accountability systems, whether through workout buddies, coaches, or online communities. External accountability can bolster discipline and foster a sense of responsibility.

3. Staying Committed to the Program:

a. Track Progress:

- **Strategy**:Regularly assess your progress. Tracking metrics, taking photos, and recording achievements can reinforce your commitment by showcasing tangible results.

b. Embrace Variety:

- **Strategy**: Introduce variety into your program to keep it engaging. This could involve trying new exercises, exploring different workout formats, or participating in diverse fitness activities.

c. Celebrate Milestones:

- **Strategy**: Acknowledge and celebrate milestones along the way. Recognizing achievements, no matter how small, reinforces the positive aspects of your fitness journey.

4. Overcoming Challenges and Setbacks:

a. Adjust Mindset:

- **Strategy**:Adopt a growth mindset. View challenges as opportunities for learning and growth rather than insurmountable obstacles. Embrace the journey as a continual process of improvement.

b. Learn from Setbacks:

- **Strategy**:Analyze setbacks objectively. Identify the root causes, learn from the experience, and use setbacks as stepping stones for future success.

c. Seek Support:

- **Strategy**: Don't hesitate to seek support during challenging times. Whether from friends, family, or professionals, a strong support system can provide encouragement and guidance.

5. Self-Care and Rest:

a. Prioritize Recovery:

- **Strategy**: Recognize the importance of rest and recovery. Overtraining can lead to burnout and increased susceptibility to setbacks. Prioritize quality sleep, active recovery, and relaxation.

b. Address Mental Health:

- **Strategy**: Mental well-being is integral to sustained commitment. If facing mental health challenges, consider seeking professional support to ensure a holistic and balanced approach to your fitness journey.

c. Reflect and Reframe:

- **Strategy**: Regularly reflect on your fitness journey. Reframe challenges as opportunities to refine your approach and develop resilience. Every setback can be a stepping stone toward greater success.

Conclusion: A Dynamic Journey of Growth

Motivation and discipline form the backbone of a successful fitness journey. By cultivating a strong sense of purpose, building consistent habits, and navigating challenges with resilience, you create a robust foundation for lasting commitment. Embrace the dynamic nature of your journey, stay adaptable, and remember that every step, whether forward or backward, contributes to your growth and ultimate success.

CHAPTER 9

Nutrition Plans for Muscle Gain: Fueling Your Strength Journey

Building muscle requires not only effective training but also a well-structured nutrition plan that supports growth and recovery. This guide outlines key principles and strategies to optimize your nutrition for muscle gain.

1. Caloric Surplus:

- **Principle**: To build muscle, you need to consume more calories than your body burns. This creates a caloric surplus, providing the energy required for muscle growth.

- **Strategy**: Calculate your daily maintenance calories and aim for a modest surplus (usually

250-500 calories per day). Track your progress and adjust caloric intake based on results.

2. Protein Intake:

- **Principle**:Protein is crucial for muscle repair and growth. Consuming an adequate amount supports protein synthesis and enhances recovery.

- **Strategy**: Aim for 1.6 to 2.2 grams of protein per kilogram of body weight. Include protein-rich foods in each meal, such as lean meats, poultry, fish, eggs, dairy, and plant-based sources like legumes and tofu.

3. Carbohydrates for Energy:

- **Principle**: Carbohydrates provide the energy necessary for intense workouts, preventing muscle breakdown for fuel.

- **Strategy**: Consume complex carbohydrates such as whole grains, fruits, vegetables, and legumes. Tailor carbohydrate intake to support energy levels during training and recovery.

4. Healthy Fats:

- **Principle**: Fats play a role in hormone production, including testosterone, which influences muscle growth. Incorporating healthy fats supports overall health and muscle-building processes.

- **Strategy**: Include sources of healthy fats such as avocados, nuts, seeds, olive oil, and fatty fish in your diet. Ensure a balanced intake without excessive amounts.

5. Nutrient Timing:

- **Principle**: Timing nutrient intake around workouts can enhance muscle protein synthesis and recovery.

- **Strategy**: Consume a balanced meal with carbohydrates and protein before and after workouts. This pre- and post-training nutrition supports energy levels and kickstarts muscle repair.

6. Hydration:

- **Principle**: Proper hydration is essential for optimal performance and recovery.

- **Strategy**: Drink water throughout the day and consider consuming fluids with electrolytes during intense workouts. Hydration aids nutrient transport and supports overall well-being.

7. Meal Frequency:

- **Principle**: Distributing your daily caloric intake across multiple meals helps sustain energy levels and promotes a steady supply of nutrients.

- **Strategy**: Aim for 4-6 smaller, balanced meals throughout the day. This approach supports continuous muscle protein synthesis.

8. Supplements:

- **Principle**: While whole foods should be your primary source of nutrients, supplements can fill gaps in your nutrition plan.

- **Strategy**:Consider supplements like whey protein, creatine, and branched-chain amino acids (BCAAs) to support muscle growth. Consult with a healthcare professional before adding supplements to your regimen.

9. Periodized Nutrition:

- **Principle**: Periodizing your nutrition involves adjusting intake based on training phases and goals.

- **Strategy**: During muscle-building phases, emphasize a slight caloric surplus and higher protein intake. Adjust nutrient ratios during cutting or maintenance phases to align with specific objectives.

10. Regular Assessments:

- **Principle**: Regularly assess your progress and adjust your nutrition plan based on results.

- **Strategy**: Track changes in muscle mass, strength gains, and overall performance. Make adjustments to caloric intake, macronutrient ratios, or meal timing as needed.

Conclusion: Tailoring Your Approach

Crafting a nutrition plan for muscle gain requires personalization based on your goals, body composition, and training regimen. Continuously assess and adjust your approach to ensure that your nutritional strategies align with your evolving needs on the journey to building strength and muscle.

Meal Prepping and Planning: A Blueprint for Nutritional Success

Efficient meal prepping and planning are foundational elements in maintaining a healthy and well-balanced diet. This guide outlines practical strategies to streamline your meal preparation, ensuring that your nutrition aligns with your goals and fits seamlessly into your lifestyle.

1. Set Clear Goals:

- **Strategy:** Define your nutritional goals, whether it's muscle gain, fat loss, or overall health. Having clear objectives will guide your meal planning choices.

2. Create a Weekly Menu:

- **Strategy**: Plan your meals for the week in advance. Include a variety of nutrient-dense foods to ensure a well-rounded diet.

3. Grocery Shopping List:

- **Strategy**: Based on your weekly menu, create a detailed grocery shopping list. This minimizes the chances of impulse purchases and ensures you have all necessary ingredients on hand.

4. Batch Cooking:

- **Strategy**: Dedicate specific days for batch cooking. Prepare larger quantities of staple foods like grains, proteins, and vegetables that can be used in multiple meals throughout the week.

5. Portion Control:

- **Strategy:** Invest in portion control containers or use a food scale to measure and divide meals into appropriate serving sizes. This aids in managing calorie intake and ensures nutritional consistency.

6. Mix and Match Ingredients:

- **Strategy**: Use versatile ingredients that can be repurposed in various ways. For example, grilled chicken can be added to salads, wraps, or stir-fries for diverse meals.

7. Pre-cut Vegetables and Fruits:

- **Strategy:** Wash, chop, and portion vegetables and fruits in advance. Having them ready-to-eat promotes healthier snacking and simplifies meal assembly.

8. Storage Solutions:

- **Strategy**: Invest in quality storage containers suitable for both refrigeration and freezing. Proper storage extends the freshness of your prepped meals.

9. Use a Meal Prep Day:

- **Strategy**: Designate a specific day for meal prepping. This focused time investment can save you hours during the week and reduce daily cooking stress.

10. Cook in Bulk:

- **Strategy**: Prepare larger quantities of certain dishes, especially those that freeze well. This creates a stockpile of convenient, ready-to-eat meals for busier days.

11. Consider Macronutrient Balance:

- **Strategy**: Aim for a balance of macronutrients (proteins, carbohydrates, and fats) in each meal.

This ensures your body receives a comprehensive array of nutrients.

12. Adapt to Your Schedule:

- **Strategy**: Tailor your meal prep routine to fit your schedule. If evenings are hectic, consider preparing breakfast and lunch in advance and cooking dinner fresh.

13. Embrace Variety:

- **Strategy**: Avoid monotony by introducing variety into your meals. Experiment with different spices, sauces, and cooking methods to keep your palate engaged.

14. Plan for Snacks:

- **Strategy:** Include healthy snacks in your meal plan to curb midday hunger. Pre-portioned snacks prevent overeating and provide a nutrient boost.

15. Review and Adjust:

- **Strategy**: Regularly assess your meal prep strategy. If certain meals are consistently left uneaten or if you find yourself lacking energy, consider adjusting your approach.

Conclusion: Sustainable Nutrition Habits

Meal prepping and planning are integral components of maintaining sustainable and healthy nutrition habits. By investing time in thoughtful preparation, you not only streamline your daily routine but also empower yourself to make nourishing food choices consistently. Adapt these strategies to your preferences and lifestyle, creating a meal prep routine that aligns seamlessly with your health and fitness goals.

Supplement Guidance: Enhancing Your Nutrition Strategically

Supplements can play a supportive role in your nutrition regimen, addressing specific needs and optimizing overall health. However, it's crucial to approach supplementation mindfully. Consult with a healthcare professional before adding any supplements to your routine. Here's a guide outlining some common supplements and their potential benefits:

1. Multivitamins:

- **Purpose**: To fill potential nutrient gaps in your diet.
- **Consideration**: Choose a high-quality multivitamin that covers essential vitamins and minerals. However, aim to obtain nutrients primarily through whole foods.

2. Omega-3 Fatty Acids:

- **Purpose**: Supports heart health, brain function, and reduces inflammation.

- **Consideration**: Sources include fatty fish (e.g., salmon), flaxseeds, and walnuts. If supplementation is necessary, choose a fish oil or algae-based omega-3 supplement.

3. Vitamin D:

- **Purpose**: Essential for bone health, immune function, and mood regulation.
- **Consideration**: Sun exposure is a natural source. If sunlight is limited, consider a vitamin D supplement, especially during winter months.

4. Protein Powders:

- **Purpose**: Convenient source of protein for muscle building and recovery.
- **Consideration**: Choose high-quality protein powders like whey, casein, or plant-based options. Use supplements to complement, not replace, whole food protein sources.

5. Creatine:

- **Purpose**: Supports energy production during high-intensity exercise, aiding muscle strength and growth.
- **Consideration**: Generally safe and well-researched. Choose a pure creatine monohydrate supplement.

6. Branched-Chain Amino Acids (BCAAs):

- **Purpose**: Aids in muscle recovery and reduces exercise-induced muscle soreness.
- **Consideration**: Found in protein-rich foods. If supplementing, choose BCAAs with a balanced ratio of leucine, isoleucine, and valine.

7. Pre-Workout Supplements:

- **Purpose**: Enhances energy, focus, and exercise performance.
- **Consideration:** Check ingredients for caffeine content and potential allergens. Use cautiously and be mindful of personal tolerance levels.

8. Iron:

- **Purpose:** Supports oxygen transport in the blood and prevents iron-deficiency anemia.
- **Consideration**: Obtain iron through dietary sources like lean meats, legumes, and leafy greens. If deficient, consult with a healthcare professional before supplementation.

9. Calcium:

- **Purpose**: Essential for bone health and muscle function.
- **Consideration**: Include dairy products, fortified plant-based milk, and leafy greens in your diet. If needed, choose a calcium supplement with vitamin D for better absorption.

10. Electrolytes:

- **Purpose:** Maintains fluid balance, supports muscle contractions, and aids in hydration.

- **Consideration**:Usually obtained through a balanced diet. Electrolyte supplements may be beneficial for intense exercise or in hot environments.

11. Probiotics:

- **Purpose**: Supports gut health and digestion.
- **Consideration**: Incorporate fermented foods like yogurt, kefir, and sauerkraut. If considering a probiotic supplement, choose one with diverse strains.

12. Fiber Supplements:

- **Purpose:** Supports digestive health and regular bowel movements.
- **Consideration:** Aim to obtain fiber from whole foods like fruits, vegetables, and whole grains. If needed, consult with a healthcare professional before adding a fiber supplement.

Conclusion: Individualized Approach

Supplement needs vary based on individual factors, diet, and health goals. Always prioritize obtaining nutrients from whole foods, and use supplements strategically to address specific deficiencies or enhance performance. Consult with a healthcare professional or a registered dietitian to ensure that supplements align with your overall health and well-being.

CHAPTER 10

Fine-Tuning Your Routine: Elevating Your Fitness Journey

Fine-tuning your fitness routine involves refining key elements to maximize effectiveness, prevent plateaus, and enhance overall well-being. Consider these strategies to optimize your approach:

1. Goal Refinement:

- **Strategy:** Reevaluate your fitness goals regularly. Ensure they are specific, measurable, achievable, relevant, and time-bound (SMART). Adjust goals as needed to stay motivated.

2. Workout Intensity:

- **Strategy:** Periodically reassess your workout intensity. Incorporate progressive overload by adjusting weights, repetitions, or workout duration to continue challenging your body.

3. Diversify Your Workouts:

- **Strategy**: Introduce variety into your routine. Include different exercises, training modalities, or activities to engage different muscle groups and prevent monotony.

4. Focus on Form:

- **Strategy**: Prioritize proper form over lifting heavier weights. Correct form reduces the risk of injury and ensures that you target the intended muscles during exercises.

5. Incorporate Functional Training:

- **Strategy**: Include exercises that mimic real-life movements. Functional training enhances overall strength and flexibility, contributing to improved daily activities and sports performance.

6. Recovery Practices:

- **Strategy:** Prioritize recovery with techniques like adequate sleep, active rest days, and stretching. Listen to your body and adjust your routine based on signs of fatigue or overtraining.

7. Nutrition Tweaks:

- **Strategy:** Fine-tune your nutrition to align with your current goals. Adjust macronutrient ratios, caloric intake, and meal timing based on your workout intensity and objectives.

8. Progressive Cardiovascular Training:

- **Strategy:** Gradually increase the intensity or duration of your cardiovascular workouts. This can involve interval training, incorporating HIIT (High-Intensity Interval Training), or progressing from steady-state to more challenging sessions.

9. Mind-Body Connection:

- **Strategy**: Cultivate mindfulness during workouts. Focus on the muscle groups being worked, your breathing, and overall body awareness. This enhances the effectiveness of each movement.

10. Regular Assessments:

- **Strategy**: Periodically assess your progress. Track changes in strength, endurance, and overall fitness. Use this information to make informed adjustments to your routine.

11. Set New Challenges:

- **Strategy**: Establish new fitness challenges periodically. This could involve achieving a specific exercise milestone, participating in an event, or mastering a new skill. Challenges keep your routine exciting and motivating.

12. Listen to Your Body:

- **Strategy:** Pay attention to signals from your body. If you experience persistent fatigue, soreness, or discomfort, consider adjusting your routine or incorporating additional rest days.

13. Consider Professional Guidance:

- **Strategy**: Consult with fitness professionals, such as personal trainers or registered dietitians, for personalized guidance. Their expertise can help fine-tune your routine to align with your goals and individual needs.

14. Goal Periodization:

- **Strategy:** Implement goal periodization. Break your fitness journey into distinct phases, each with specific objectives. This approach allows you to focus on different aspects of fitness over time.

15. Enjoy the Process:

- **Strategy**: Embrace the joy of movement and the process of self-improvement. Enjoying your workouts fosters a positive mindset, making it more likely that you'll stay consistent with your routine.

Conclusion: A Dynamic Fitness Journey

Fine-tuning your fitness routine is an ongoing process that adapts to your evolving goals and needs. By incorporating these strategies, you create a dynamic and effective fitness journey that promotes long-term success and well-being.

Incorporating Advanced Exercises: Elevating Your Workout Routine

As you progress in your fitness journey, introducing advanced exercises can add complexity, challenge different muscle groups, and take your workouts to the next level. Here are some illustrative examples of advanced exercises to incorporate into your routine:

1. Plyometric Exercises:

Exercise: Box Jumps

Illustration: Start by standing in front of a sturdy box or platform. Bend your knees and explode upward, landing softly on the box. Step back down and repeat.

Benefits: Enhances explosive power, agility, and lower body strength.

2. Olympic Lifts:

Exercise: Clean and Jerk

Illustration: Begin with a barbell on the ground. Perform a clean (lifting the bar to shoulder height) followed by a jerk (pressing the bar overhead). Ensure proper form and controlled movements.

Benefits: Targets multiple muscle groups, improves coordination, and promotes full-body strength.

3. Advanced Core Exercises:

Exercise: Hanging Leg Raises

Illustration: Hang from a pull-up bar and lift your legs straight up towards the ceiling, engaging your core muscles. Lower your legs with control to complete one repetition.

Benefits: Targets the lower abdominal muscles and enhances overall core strength.

4. Unilateral Exercises:

Exercise: Bulgarian Split Squats

Illustration: Stand facing away from a bench with one foot elevated behind you. Lower your body into a lunge position, ensuring the front knee doesn't go past the toes.

Benefits: Improves balance, targets each leg individually, and activates stabilizing muscles.

5. Bodyweight Strength:

Exercise: One-Arm Push-Ups

Illustration: Assume a push-up position and shift your weight to one side, allowing one hand to come off the ground. Lower your chest towards the floor and push back up.

Benefits: Increases chest and triceps strength while challenging stability.

6. Mobility and Flexibility:

Exercise: Turkish Get-Up

Illustration: Lie on your back holding a kettlebell. Perform a series of movements to stand up while keeping the kettlebell overhead. Reverse the sequence to return to the starting position.
Benefits: Enhances full-body mobility, stability, and coordination.

7. Suspension Training:

Exercise: TRX Rows

Illustration: Set up TRX straps at chest height. Hold the handles, lean back, and perform a rowing motion. Adjust your body angle to modify the resistance.

Benefits: Targets the back muscles and improves stability through an adjustable resistance range.

8. Advanced Cardiovascular Exercise:

Exercise: Burpee Pull-Ups

Illustration: Start with a burpee, then jump up and perform a pull-up. Land softly and repeat the sequence.

Benefits: Combines strength and cardio elements for an efficient full-body workout.

9. Stability Ball Exercises:

Exercise: Stability Ball Pike

Illustration: Assume a plank position with your feet on a stability ball. Lift your hips towards the ceiling, rolling the ball towards your hands. Return to the starting position.

Benefits: Engages the core and stabilizing muscles, improving balance and strength.

10. Agility Drills:

Exercise: Ladder Drills

Illustration: Use an agility ladder for various footwork patterns, such as high knees, side shuffles, or quick steps.

Benefits: Enhances agility, coordination, and cardiovascular endurance.

Conclusion: Safely Progressing Your Fitness Journey

Incorporating advanced exercises requires a foundation of strength, stability, and proper form. Progress gradually, ensuring mastery of fundamental movements before attempting more complex exercises. Consult with a fitness professional if needed to ensure safety and effectiveness in your advanced workout routine.

Personalizing the Program for Long-Term Success: Tailoring Your Fitness Journey

Personalizing your fitness program is key to sustained success. Consider these personalized strategies to make your routine effective, enjoyable, and adaptable for long-term commitment:

1. Identify Your Personal Goals:

- **Strategy:** Clarify your specific fitness goals, whether it's weight loss, muscle gain, improved endurance, or overall well-being.

2. Assess Your Current Fitness Level:

- **Strategy:** Evaluate your current fitness capabilities, considering strength, flexibility, cardiovascular health, and any specific areas for improvement.

3. Consider Your Preferences:

- **Strategy**: Incorporate activities you enjoy. Whether it's dancing, hiking, or weightlifting, choosing enjoyable exercises increases adherence.

4. Tailor Your Routine to Your Lifestyle:

- **Strategy**: Align your workout schedule with your daily routine. Choose workout times that fit seamlessly into your day to ensure consistency.

5. Integrate Variety:

- **Strategy**: Embrace diversity in your workouts. Include a mix of strength training, cardiovascular exercises, flexibility work, and activities that challenge balance and coordination.

6. Listen to Your Body:

- **Strategy**: Pay attention to how your body responds to different exercises and intensities. Adjust your program based on your body's signals and recovery needs.

7. Progress Gradually:

- **Strategy:** Incrementally increase the intensity and complexity of your workouts. This gradual approach reduces the risk of burnout and minimizes the chance of injury.

8. Adapt to Changing Goals:

- **Strategy:** Periodically reassess your goals and adjust your program accordingly. As your fitness level improves, your goals may evolve.

9. Include Active Recovery:

- **Strategy:** Integrate active recovery days into your routine. This might involve light activities like walking, yoga, or swimming to aid in muscle recovery.

10. Incorporate Periodization:

- **Strategy**: Implement periodization principles by cycling through phases of different training intensities. This approach prevents plateauing and promotes continuous improvement.

11. Explore New Activities:

- **Strategy:** Keep your routine fresh by trying new sports or activities. This not only adds excitement but also engages different muscle groups.

12. Establish a Support System:

- **Strategy:** Surround yourself with a supportive network. This might include workout buddies, fitness communities, or professionals who can provide guidance.

13. Prioritize Recovery:

- **Strategy**: Allocate time for adequate rest and recovery. Quality sleep, proper nutrition, and stress management are integral components of long-term success.

14. Set Realistic Expectations:

- **Strategy**: Establish achievable short-term and long-term goals. Realistic expectations foster a positive mindset and prevent discouragement.

15. Consult with Professionals:

- **Strategy**: Seek guidance from fitness professionals, including personal trainers and nutritionists, to create a program tailored to your individual needs and goals.

Conclusion: A Sustainable Fitness Journey

Personalizing your fitness program ensures that it aligns with your unique attributes and goals, making it more likely to be enjoyable and sustainable in the long run. Regularly reassess and adapt your routine to keep it challenging and engaging, promoting continuous progress on your fitness journey.

CHAPTER 11

Celebrating Success, Reflecting on Achievements, and Setting New Fitness Goals: A Holistic Approach to Your Fitness Journey

1. Celebrating Success:

Strategy: Take a moment to acknowledge and celebrate your achievements, no matter how small. Recognizing milestones boosts motivation and reinforces a positive mindset.

Example: Whether it's reaching a weight loss goal, lifting a heavier weight, or consistently completing your workouts, celebrate with a small reward, such as treating yourself to a healthy meal or enjoying a relaxing activity.

2. Reflecting on Achievements:

Strategy: Reflect on the progress you've made since the beginning of your fitness journey. Consider both physical and mental transformations, acknowledging the positive changes in your overall well-being.

Example: Journal about your fitness journey, noting improvements in strength, stamina, and mood. Capture how these changes have positively impacted your daily life and mindset.

3. Setting New Fitness Goals:

Strategy: Evaluate your current fitness goals and consider what new objectives you'd like to pursue. Set SMART goals (Specific, Measurable, Achievable, Relevant, Time-bound) to guide your next phase of progress.

Example: If you've achieved a weight loss goal, you might set a new goal focused on building muscle strength or improving flexibility. Ensure your goals align with your evolving priorities.

4. Creating a Vision Board:

Strategy: Develop a vision board that visually represents your fitness goals. Include images or quotes that inspire and motivate you, serving as a constant reminder of what you're working towards.

Example: Cut out pictures of activities, physique goals, or fitness quotes that resonate with your aspirations. Place the vision board where you'll see it regularly.

5. Joining a Fitness Community:

Strategy: Connect with a fitness community, either online or locally. Sharing your achievements and goals with like-minded individuals provides support and fosters a sense of camaraderie.

Example: Participate in fitness challenges, engage in discussions, and celebrate milestones within the community. The shared enthusiasm can be contagious and inspiring.

6. **Periodic Assessments**:

Strategy: Schedule regular assessments to track your progress. These assessments can include fitness tests, body measurements, or performance evaluations.

Example: Set specific intervals, such as every three months, to assess your fitness metrics. Use the results to adjust your goals and training program accordingly.

7. **Incorporating New Activities:**

Strategy: Keep your fitness routine dynamic by incorporating new activities or sports. Trying something different not only challenges your body but also adds an element of excitement.

Example: If you've been primarily focused on weight training, consider adding activities like yoga, cycling, or swimming to diversify your workouts.

8. Personalizing Challenges:

Strategy: Create personalized fitness challenges to keep things interesting. These challenges could be related to endurance, strength, or skill development.

Example: Challenge yourself to run a certain distance within a set time frame, master a new exercise, or achieve a specific number of consecutive push-ups.

9. Establishing Habitual Practices:

Strategy: Develop habits that support your fitness journey, such as consistent sleep patterns, mindful eating, and stress management. These habits contribute to overall well-being.

Example: Implement a regular sleep schedule, practice mindful eating by savoring each meal, and incorporate stress-reducing activities like meditation or nature walks.

10. Seeking Professional Guidance:

Strategy: Consult with fitness professionals, including personal trainers or nutritionists, to refine your goals and receive expert advice on optimizing your fitness program.

Example: A trainer can help design a personalized workout plan, offer guidance on nutrition, and provide ongoing support to ensure you stay on track.

Conclusion: Embracing the Journey

Celebrating success, reflecting on achievements, and setting new fitness goals create a continuous and fulfilling cycle in your fitness journey. Embrace the evolving nature of your goals, savor your accomplishments, and approach each new phase with enthusiasm and determination. Your fitness journey is a dynamic and transformative experience—enjoy every step of it!

CHAPTER 12

Appendices

1. Exercise Glossary:
- A comprehensive guide to the exercises mentioned in the book, including detailed instructions and illustrations to ensure proper form and technique.

2. Workout Logs:
- Printable workout logs to help you track your progress, set goals, and stay organized throughout your bodybuilding journey.

3. Nutritional Charts:
- Charts outlining macronutrient content, portion sizes, and nutritional information for common foods, aiding in meal planning and dietary management.

4. Goal Setting Worksheets:

- Practical worksheets to assist you in defining and refining your fitness goals, ensuring they are SMART and align with your aspirations.

Additional Resources

1. **Recommended Reading**:
   - A curated list of books, articles, and research papers on bodybuilding, nutrition, and overall fitness to deepen your understanding and stay informed.

2. **Online Platforms and Communities:**
   - Links to reputable websites, forums, and social media groups where you can connect with fellow fitness enthusiasts, seek advice, and share your experiences.

3. **Podcasts and Webinars:**
   - Recommendations for podcasts and webinars featuring experts in the field of bodybuilding,

providing valuable insights, tips, and discussions.

4. Fitness Apps and Tools:

- An overview of popular fitness apps and tools that can assist you in tracking workouts, monitoring nutrition, and staying motivated on your fitness journey.

VERY IMPORTANT TOOL

5. Ultimate body building picture illustration book

A book by same Author "me".

Giving pictorial illustrations on body building techniques mentioned in this very book and also the meals highlighted.

Frequently Asked Questions

1. How often should I change my workout routine?

- Explore the importance of workout variety and the factors that influence when and how to modify your exercise regimen for optimal results.

2. What role does sleep play in bodybuilding?

- Understand the crucial connection between quality sleep, muscle recovery, and overall performance in the context of bodybuilding.

3. How can I prevent workout plateaus?

- Learn strategies to overcome plateaus, including progressive overload, periodization, and the incorporation of advanced training techniques.

4. Is supplementation necessary for bodybuilding?

- Explore the role of supplements, their potential benefits, and considerations for incorporating them into your nutrition plan.

5. What's the ideal balance between cardio and strength training?

- Gain insights into the synergy between cardiovascular exercise and strength training, helping you strike an effective balance for your fitness goals.

6. How do I stay motivated during challenging periods?

- Discover practical tips for maintaining motivation, setting realistic expectations, and overcoming challenges on your bodybuilding journey.

7. Can bodybuilding be adapted for different fitness levels?

- Learn how bodybuilding principles can be tailored to accommodate beginners, intermediate, and advanced fitness levels, ensuring inclusivity and progression.

8. How do I prevent injuries while bodybuilding?

- Explore injury prevention strategies, including proper warm-ups, cooldowns, and form checks, to prioritize safety during your workouts.

NOTE: The appendices, additional resources, and frequently asked questions are designed to complement the content of "Ultimate Proper Body Building" and provide valuable tools and information for a holistic and informed bodybuilding experience.

DON'T FORGET THE VERY IMPORTANT ILLUSTRATIVE BOOK BY FRANK C MOORE. THAT MAKES YOU COMPLETELY FIT.